CW01283385

Everyone's eczema story is different. As a health coach I have heard very similar eczema stories. Most clients tell me it started for them as a baby then appeared off and on again during their life. When they reached their mid-twenties it flared up majorly which is when they usually seek me out for help. Other clients have had it non-stop for their whole lives. Some cases are far more unusual and their first time having eczema was in adulthood. For me, I had it since I was a child. My first big flare up was when I was four. I had a birthday party at this super cool jungle gym with all of my friends. My parents told me it didn't seem to break my spirits but I had eczema all over my arms, legs, and back. At that time they thought it was just a rash...

ECZEMA HEALING

LIFESTYLE TRANSFORMATION

Michelle Mills

INTRODUCTION
Let's Transform Your Life

Welcome to your new life. I am very excited that you have chosen to heal your eczema naturally. This book will teach you how to live a non-toxic life that will help you get rid of your eczema and prevent other diseases later in life. Humanity has grown farther and farther from nature and as a result we have created lifestyles that are not only bad for our environment but bad for our bodies. You will learn how to adjust your diet, detox your home, get better sleep, and become friends with your gut bacteria.

This book will introduce you to me, Michelle Mills, who is a certified health coach dedicated to helping you heal your eczema. After reading this book if you ever have a question or two please feel free to contact me via email: coachmichellemills@gmail.com. If you would like emotional support to help you cope with your skin then you might be interested in my facbook group: Healthy Skin Happy Living. This is a group full of people from all over the world who are on this healing journey, just like you. You will find that the members of this group are in all stages of eczema all with unique stories and situations. I created it so my eczema friends wouldn't feel isolated in society. I also interact often in this group to answer your questions. I hope you enjoy this book and find that you start to heal very quickly!

My Story

Everyone's eczema story is different. As a health coach I have heard very similar eczema stories. Most clients tell me it started for them as a baby then appeared off and on again during their life. When they reached their mid-twenties it flared up majorly which is when they usually seek me out for help. Other clients have had it non-stop for their whole lives. Some cases are far more unusual and their first time having eczema was in adulthood. For me, I had it since I was a child. My first big flare up was when I was four. I had a birthday party at this super cool jungle gym with all of my friends. My parents told me it didn't seem to break my spirits but I had eczema all over my arms, legs, and back. At that time they thought it was just a rash.

Two years later I had my second big flare up and was diagnosed with dyshidrotic eczema. I was prescribed bactroban, a cortisol topical steroid. I remember quite vividly that I had rashes on my hands that would crack and bleed. It was pretty embarrassing because neither teachers nor my peers understood what was happening with me.

What is Wrong With Me?

My parents thought I was allergic to oak trees because logically to them I would have little outbreaks of eczema only during the fall and they thought the trees might be producing pollen that was bothering me. I recall this one time for a science project we went outside to examine leaves and I couldn't participate because it included touching oak leaves. Imagine one of your classmates telling the teacher they can't be outside because their hands have a weird rash on them from tree pollen. Of course my classmates thought I was a bit strange. I was totally embarrased and felt as though I was the weird kid "allergic" to trees. This demonstrates not only how confusing eczema is

My Story

to the person with it but also to their loved ones.

Years later in middle school I had the worst of the worst. My legs were absolutely covered. Like many people, I couldn't help but itch the spots in my sleep which led to oozing, bleeding spores all over. Unfortunately I have this very vivid memory of being in gym class and having to wear shorts. I wasn't a very self-conscious kid so when people would ask me what was on my legs I would just explain it was eczema. But! There was this one time when I felt the infected areas oozing down my legs. I couldn't take it and I didn't feel as though other people should have to look at my legs so I ended up having to change back into my jeans and sit out for the day. This was also the time in my life that I would wake up with my legs stuck to the sheets waiting for me to peel them off the dried blood and ooze. I apologize for the graphic nature of this section but for those with severe eczema, I know you understand. I was able to treat this by applying a topical steroid then wrapping my legs in plastic wrap while I slept. This was incredibly uncomfortable but worked. I was very lucky to not go through extreme TSW (topical steroid withdrawal) and this is because I used the cream pretty sparingly.

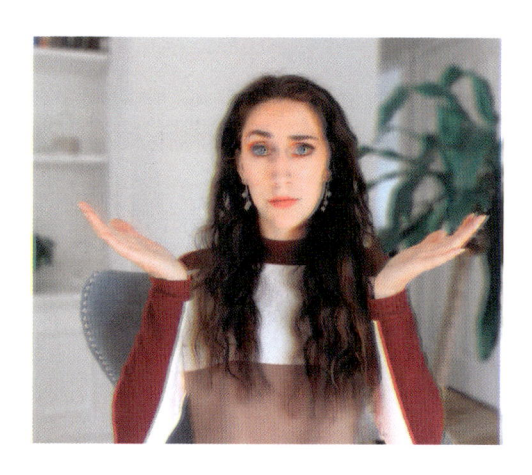

Since then I have got a few patches on my legs and arms. The flare-ups were always temporary and didn't cause me much harm. I would have

My Story

at least one dry spot on the back of my knee pretty much constantly. I remember I signed to a modeling agency in May of 2017 and of course I had some eczema on my arm. I was sitting outside in my car before my meeting to sign with the agency. I thought to myself "Oh no, I wonder if they will notice my eczema. Will this make them not want to sign me?" I actually ended up putting powder foundation on the flare-up to reduce the redness. I think that worked because the agency didn't notice.

Welcome to September 2017

This story is the whole reason I am writing this book. I had just gone through a pretty emotional time in my life and I did what I usually do, emotionally ate. I was eating a pint of ice cream nearly weekly. I was eating cheese and bagels and all sorts of things that was very unlike me. Up until this point I had been paleo-based for about two years. I actually had completed the Whole30 in that June but in July relapsed into bad habits quickly after because of how rebellious I felt. In August, I made a pretty huge move to another state. I am setting the scene for how most people end up with a horrible eczema flare up. Poor eating habits added with stress equals eczema.

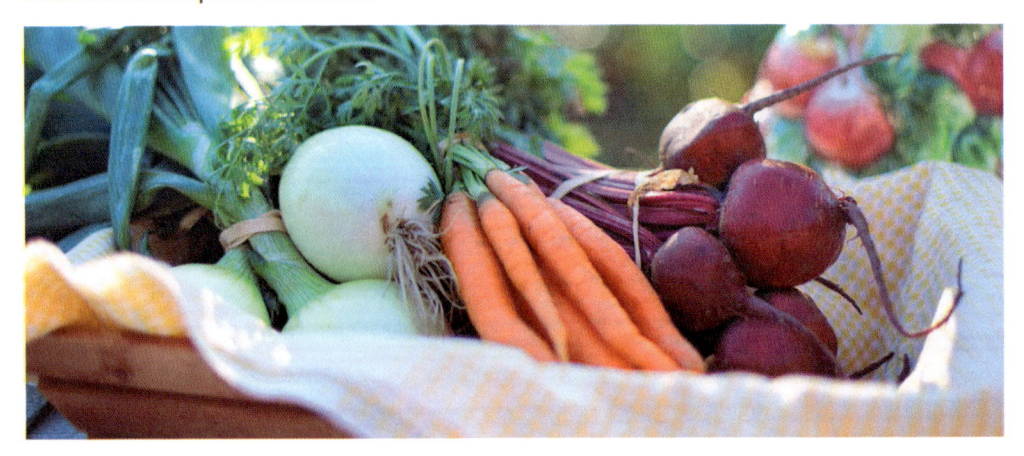

My Story

It started with a pretty harmless patch on the inside of my elbow. It kept growing everyday into a larger and larger patch. It then popped up on the inside of my other elbow and the backs of my knees. It started to worry me because it began to feel very dry and itchy. At the time I had no idea what I know now about how to heal your skin from the inside out. I continued to eat my weekly pint of ice cream and bagels at work. The patches became embarrassing and started to impact my social life. I really wished to wear long sleeves to hide the patches but as it got worse I no longer could bear the feeling of anything touching my skin. I hit my breaking point December 16th, 2017. On the previous day it was my dad's birthday. My family all went over to my nana's house for dinner. It was a really nice meal and to my surprise my nana had made a cheesecake for dessert. Cheesecake used to be one of my biggest weaknesses. My dad and I enjoyed shared a piece of cheesecake that night. The very next day I was in the worst shape of my life. My arms flared up in the brightest red painful eczema I have ever had.

Finally Healing

By Late December of 2017 my flare-up grew from a few patches to taking over my arms, reaching my hands, and breakouts on my legs. I have honestly never been in more pain in my whole life. The worst part was healthy foods like berries and spinach were causing me the most pain (this is from salicylates which you will learn about later)! Through tons of trial and error I learned what foods allowed me to control my eczema symptoms. From that point forward I had to learn why certain chemical compounds in foods cause eczema. I dove in and ended up doing so much research that I fully learned to the cellular level why people develop eczema.

My Story

By March 2018, I had control over my skin again, and I finally felt like myself! In the end, this flare-up was a huge blessing and I learned so much. In the process of managing my eczema I started helping a few people that found my story on the internet and guess what, they healed too. After seeing their skin transform, it dawned on me that I was really helping people. I knew for a fact that becoming a health coach would let me reach more people. I want nothing more than to guide people through transitioning to healthy lifestyles that result in less pain, and more living. So let's get healthy together! This is a comprehensive guide on how to get you (or your family member) to not only have clear skin but to establish a healthy lifesytle as well.

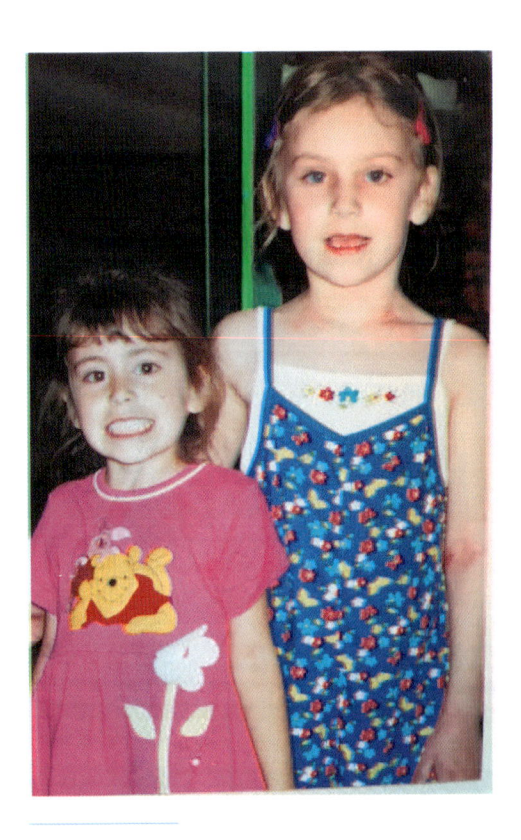

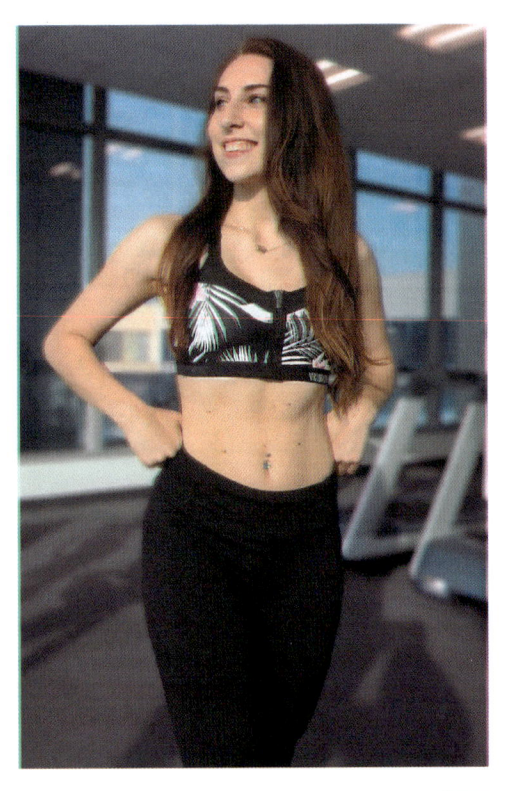

What is Eczema

Eczema is an autoimmune disorder. Interestingly, eczema has very little to do with the skin itself. Instead it has everything to do with the health of the body, specifically your gut, liver, and immune system. Autoimmune disorders usually develop from leaky gut. Leaky gut, also known as intestinal permeability, is when your diet, lifestyle, and environment cause tears in your gut lining. Our gut lining is only one cell thick which is pretty worrisome if you ask me. We have to keep up our gut health and keep the lining healthy. Leaky gut is reversible which is great news. That is why most autoimmune disorders can heal.

When your intestines have tears it allows bacteria, food particles, and toxins to enter your bloodstream. Why is this a problem? Our bodies are fantastic at managing our well being. The body has a system in place that acts like an army. There is something called antibodies which act as scouts. They make sure that there are no enemies lurking around. When we have unknown substances in our bloodstream, the antibodies mark them as harmful. The part of our immune system that goes into battle are our killer cells. This is where eczema differs from psoriasis.

We have many types of killer cells but autoimmune disorders and diseases are characterized by TH1 and TH2 killer cells. For example eczema is a TH2 dominant autoimmune disorder but psoriasis is TH1. I realize this probably means very little to you but the point is, it is important to understand that eczema has a root cause. It has very little to do with the skin itself and it has to be repaired from the inside-out.

Now that you know that eczema is a TH2 dominant disorder you can avoid certain substances that will create a further dominance such as coffee. You will read more about this in the diet section of this book. Get ready, you are about to learn a lot! Congrats again on your healing journey.

Stages of Eczema

What are the stages of eczema healing? I will teach you how to gauge where you are in your journey. Some of you may have severe painful eczema and others may have a few patches here or there. This protocol was designed around months of research on what eczema is and how it is effected by foods, environment, and stress.

Some of you reading may even have TSW which is short for topical steroid withdrawal. This occurs when you come off of strong topical steroids or prolonged use of them. The skin will go through cycles to detox from the steroids which show as very dry and red skin over and over throughout the span of about a year. The skin will often ooze a foul smelling liquid. Luckily this process can be shortened through an antioxidant rich diet.

Stage 1

This is the worst of the worst. This is for those who lose sleep because they are in pain. You are in stage one if:

1. Eczema is located in more than one spot on your body. You may have very large flare-ups on one part and smaller ones on another part of your body.
2. It is considerably red in color.
3. You often feel a burning and/or stinging sensation.
4. It is sensitive to the touch. This may mean it hurts while wearing tight clothes or clothes made from irritating materials such as wool.
5. You are going through TSW (topical steroid withdrawal)

Stage 2

It is good news if you are in stage two but you are not in the clear. If you do not quickly change your habits it could make a turn for the worst and fall into stage 1. On the other hand stage 2 can also go to stage 3 quickly as well.

Stages of Eczema

1. Your flareup has turned mostly into a white, pink, or flesh color.
2. You have smaller patches than before
3. Itchiness has reduced from everyday to a few times a week.
4. Your skin may be raised and look like hives. If it is also more pink than skin tone then be careful you could dip into stage 1 fast.
5. For TSW you are seeing lots of flakiness and dryness.

Stage 3

Congrats! This is the easiest to heal but the stage you will most likely remain in the longest. This stage could last up to a year depending on how closely you avoid triggering foods.

1. For lighter skin tones, the skin might be discolored lighter than your skin. For darker, it may be darker. Some patches may just be skin color.
2. Any pink patches are around the size of a quarter
3. You rarely feel itchy. If you do, it is mild.
4. You feel better. Your eczema is manageable and not affecting social life.
5. For TSW the flareups have minimized in size.

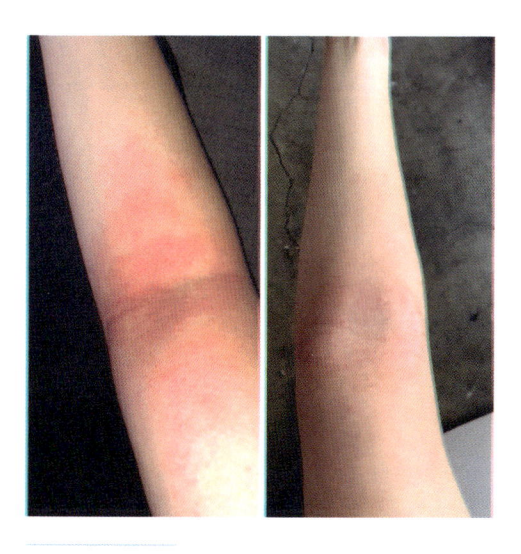

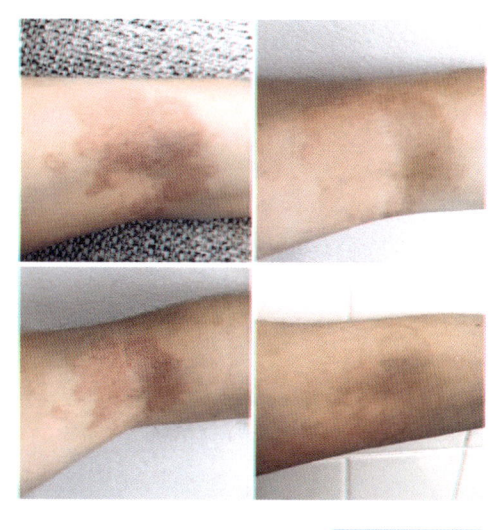

Diet Intro

Now it is time to start healing! Please glance at the blue chart to the right. This chart shows you which foods to completely avoid while you are healing your eczema. This applies to ALL stages! Good luck on your journey and remember: "As human beings, we are science." We are comprised of molecules that interact with other molecules, some of which harm us.

Eczema is not a skin problem, it is a full body issue that must be healed from the inside, out.

The Worst

These foods are likely the main reason you developed eczema to begin with if your eczema is diet related. I suggest reading ingredient labels if you chose to eat packaged food because manufacturers love to sneak these ingredients into many, many products.

The safest way to approach eczema healing is by eating foods that only have one ingredient like vegetables. This means no more cakes, bread, ice cream, or yogurt unless you can find them without "FREDG foods". This isn't as difficult as it sounds. I am able to find cashew based yogurt, coconut ice cream, and nut-based cheeses. Once you get into stage 3, check out my website for some sweet treats that are free of these harmful ingredients!

Gut Harming

Egg whites contain an enzyme called lysozyme. Numerous research studies show that this enzyme eats through the intestine lining (leaky gut). Gut health is at the center of healing. The protein gluten and the sugar lactose will also dig through the gut lining. The gut can be repaired! Be patient.

Think of your gut like a cut on your knee. Each time you add a toxin into your life, for example stress, this cut gets worse. We do not expect our cuts to heal in a week so neither will our eczema.

Immune System Harming

While there is need for more research (as of 2018), I have personally tested all of these and found that they drastically impaired my immune system. Red grapes contain an antioxidant called resveratrol that is very

Diet Intro

THE FOUNDATION
THE WORST "FREDG Foods"
1. Fried foods
2. Refined sugar (white sugar, brown sugar, beet sugar)
3. Eggs
4. Dairy (yogurt, milk, butter, cheeses)
5. Gluten (wheat, rye, barley, etc.)

IMMUNE SYSTEM HARMING
Caffeine (coffee, green tea, black tea, chocolate)
Red grapes/Red wine
Turmeric
Cumin
Curry

GUT HARMING
Gluten
Eggs (specifically egg whites)
Lactose

BAD FOR HEALTH IN GENERAL
Trans-fats
High fructose corn syrup

CAUSES INFLAMMATION
Canola/Rapeseed oil
Sunflower oil
Safflower oil
Corn oil
Carrageenan

beneficial for those WITHOUT eczema. For those with eczema, it further creates a TH2 dominance which slows down eczema healing. Turmeric, cumin, and curry contain the antioxidant called curcumin which has the same affects as resveratrol. The same goes for caffeine as well. Make sure if you drink tea, it is an herbal decaffeinated tea.

Make sure to review the "Bad for Health in General" and "Causes Inflammation" lists. The oils that cause inflammation and the ingredients that are bad for health are found in countless processed foods. Try an experiment when you go to a store like Target. Go to their ice cream section and grab a Ben & Jerry's ice cream pint. Read the ingredients list and try to identify any ingredients you think would help heal your gut. You will be shocked to see that there may only be 1 which would be water.

Become a label reading genius. I have trained myself for years so now I can scan a product's ingredients list and know in 2 seconds if it's for me!

Diet

Let's talk FREDG (pronounced fridge) foods. This is my acronym to help you remember which foods to avoid indefinitely. F stands for fried foods, R for refined sugar, E for eggs, D for dairy, and G for gluten. If you can identify that your skin reacts badly to eating then avoiding these should really help. Start making these changes immediately. When I knew nothing about healing eczema, I unknowingly was eating precisely the wrong foods for healing. For most people eggs seem like a perfectly healthy snack. I ate them nearly everyday until I started researching foods to create a diet that heals eczema **quickly**. That research showed me that an enzyme in egg whites called lysozyme creates leaky gut (also called intestinal permeability).

My occasional bagel as a snack, brie cheese on crackers, and 4 eggs for breakfast was the exact recipe to cause eczema. When I finally cut out cheese I ended up eating healthy vegetables like spinach and carrots. Does this sound like you? One night in the peak of my painful eczema journey, I was snacking on some healthy carrots. During my sleep (30 minutes later) I was awoken by horrible itching pain. I was so upset and confused because I thought my healthy snack was going to help me, not hurt me. This my friends, was a reaction to a plant chemical called salicylates which showed me that my liver was overworked.

Avoiding FREDG foods is just the foundation to get on a healthy journey. I developed an in-depth diet that speeds up the healing process. It was created through extensive research on eczema and how to heal it from the inside out. There are a lot of diets out there. Some people swear by the vegan diet and others find that eating mostly meat helps. From my experience, those diets are good at very **slowly** reducing eczema.

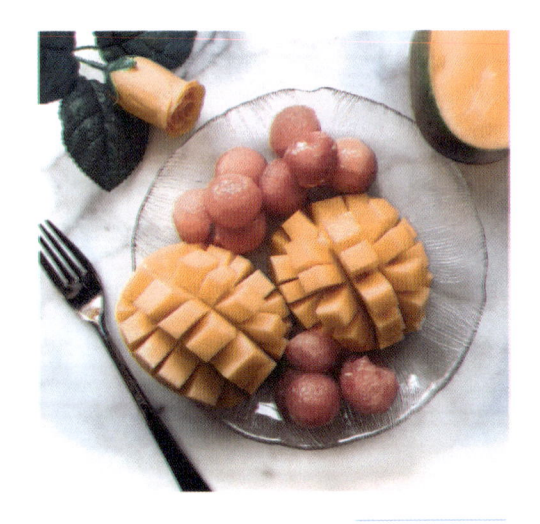

Eczema Healing Lifestyle Transformation ©
by Michelle Mills

Diet

I have designed a diet that heals eczema very quickly by balancing the immune system, healing leaky gut, and detoxing the liver called The Gut Healing Eczema Protocol. However, I currently only offer this diet through my coaching programs. This diet shouldn't be blindly followed without instruction.

Optimally I would work with every individual 1-on-1 to adjust the diet based on prior allergies, stress levels, and mental health. The diet is broken up into the 6 steps where step 1 is the most healing for severe eczema. Following along with the stages of eczema listed in this book, this would be stage 1.

Stage 1 causes the most aggravation in the day to day life. You often are very itchy, lose sleep, and feel generally uncomfortable daily. The diet for stage 1 is a very specific and limited diet that works to reduce itching and start to clear up the skin. It is designed to heal the gut by giving us our most healing foods first like bone broth, leeks, cabbage, and celery.

You reach stage 2 when the skin begins to clear up and you can start to eat a larger range of foods. Stage 3 is potentially the longest stage but the most comfortable to live with. Stage 3 lasts one year and you can pretty much each all healthy clean foods.

Once the year is over you should be able to accidentally consume a FREDG foods and not see a visible reaction. However, let me be clear, you cannot go back to eating a poor diet again. But you should see this as a blessing not a curse. By avoiding harmful foods you are preventing serious diseases later in life like heart disease, cancer, and diabetes.

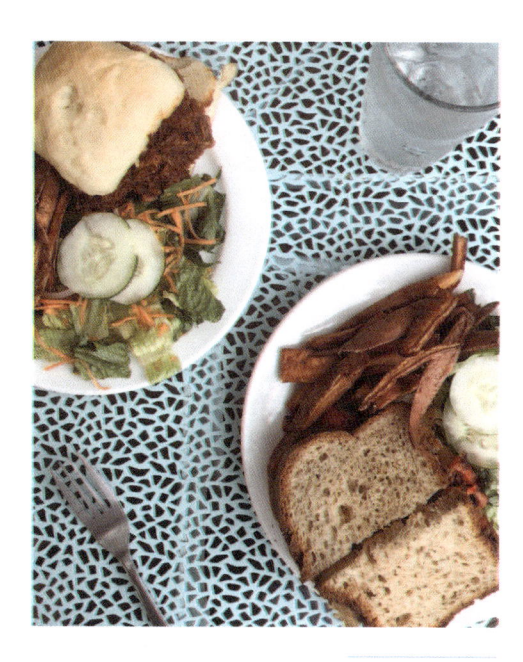

Supplements

Supplements can be used while you have a flare-up to promote healing. Supplements are a tricky topic and it is important that you consult your doctor before starting to take any new supplements. There are certain conditions where supplements may interfere with medications. As long as it is approved by your doctor I am excited to tell you all about the healing properties of these specific supplements.

Probiotics

This is something that absolutely everyone should be taking. Probiotics add good bacteria back to your gut which helps with mood regulation, nutrient absorption, and fighting off bad bacteria. There are many strains of bacteria that are found in probiotics.

Research shows that Lactobacillus Rhamnosus is a particular strain of bacteria that is especially beneficial for eczema. I recommend that you find a probiotic that includes that strain, contains a broad range of other bacteria, and is in the billions. Probiotic supplements will tell you on the front of the bottle how much of the bacteria is in them. Making sure it is in the billions will ensure that the bacteria makes it to the gut. Bacteria is sensitive to chemicals and heat and often times gets killed off before it reaches the gut. You also should make sure to buy the probiotics from the refridgerator section and store them in your fridge at home. Garden of Life brand has an innovative bottle that keeps the bacteria alive which is perfectly fine as well.

Glycine

This is my favorite supplement for healing. It is an amino acid which is a building block of proteins. I recommend taking it every night before bed because it helps you get good rest. Glycine helps relieve an extreme itch attack. I have not been able to understand biologically why this works but I have tested it myself and with my clients.

When I had eczema for the last time, I had the worst flare-up of my life. I was shopping around a cute little town not far from my own. I went to a coffee shop and bought a gluten-free brownie. After that, I shopped around a local grocery store to find some eczema safe

Supplements

goodies. When I got into the car to return home I started eating the brownie. Fifteen minutes later, while I was driving, I had a massive itch attack. My skin flared bright red and I was so itchy it was painful.

I remember calling my mom screaming and crying because I was in so much pain. I didn't know what I was going to do. When I finally made it home I took a glycine because I wanted to just take a nap. Amazingly, within 5 minutes I felt so much better. It is not magic and doesn't heal eczema by itself but glycine is so effective at managing itch attacks like that one.

L-glutamine & L-lysine

These two supplements are amino acids just like glycine but they function differently. Research shows that L-glutamine repairs the gut lining. However, research also shows that prolonged use of L-glutamine produces glutamate which is a neurotoxin. You are likely to experience brain fog and learning issues if you are exposed to glutamate too long. This is new research as of 2019 but it is important for you all to be aware of it. Because of the healing properties of l-glutamine for the gut, I recommend taking it for the first two weeks of healing. After that switch to l-lysine which works great as well. During my healing, I had prolonged use of l-glutamine (about 6 months) and was perfectly fine. As research progresses I will be updating you all on my YouTube channel.

The safest method might be to only take l-lysine from the beginning. I recommend taking it with lunch. If you need help creating a supplement schedule I have many videos on my YouTube channel already to help you out!

Vitamin D

Later on in this book, you will learn more about vitamin D in the "Vital Nutrients" section. Vitamin D is critical for healing. I recommend taking vitamin D with lunch. It is best absorbed in the afternoon. Try not to take it before bed because it can make you feel energized. As you progress on your healing journey you will take less and less supplements. Leaky gut can prevent the body from properly absorbing nutrients. During healing our bodies will use

Supplements

up more nutrients than normal. As you start to heal you can wean yourself off of the supplements. Now that I am healed I only take probiotics daily and take vitamin D during the winter when I cannot get the proper amount of sunlight. If you live in a dark/cold country try taking vitamin D year round.

Milk Thistle

This is another magic supplement. Milk Thistle is a herb that naturally detoxes the liver. Why does your liver have anything to do with eczema? If you have ever eaten something healthy and wondered why you developed an itch-attack your liver is the reason.

The liver's primary function is to remove toxins from your body and becomes very overworked from your diet and lifestyle. One of the duties of your liver is to protect your body from natural chemicals that plants have. One chemical is called salicylates which are natural insecticides.

An example of fruit high in salicylates is pineapples. To help heal your liver you should avoid produce that contains this chemical. While you do this, it is important to take milk thistle to aid your liver. Be sure not to use milk thistle for longer than 3 months because it can lead to a lazy liver.

Candida Enzymes

The brand that is particularly amazing is called Candex which is linked from my shop on my website! This supplement uses cellulase and hemicellulase to break apart the candida bacteria cells. An enzyme's job is to break down larger things into smaller things. For example our bodies use lipase to break down lipids aka fats. Candida is very common for people with eczema and causes severe sugar cravings. The reason why is because the bacteria feeds off of sugar.

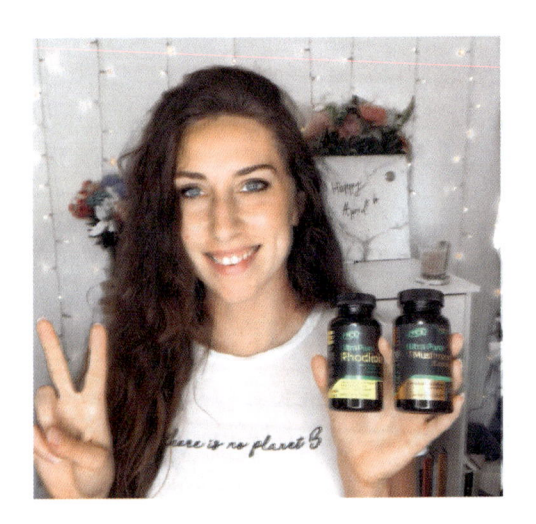

Eczema Healing Lifestyle Transformation © by Michelle Mills

www.coachmichellemills.com

Moisturizing

What should you use to moisturize? This will differ slightly from person to person. I have learned from my clients that some people can use coconut oil and see great results and some people see a decline in their skin. You will have to test different combinations but the best I have found is shea butter mixed with geranium essential oils.

As long as the oil or butter is natural you should see good results. Another combination that worked well for me for itching is olive oil mixed with a few drops of tea tree oil. Make sure to be checking the ingredients on any package you buy. You may believe you are buying just shea butter but find toxic chemicals like fragrance.

What we put on our skin is just as important as what we put inside our bodies. Our skin absorbs most of what we apply to our skin whether it's toxic chemicals or vitamin e from healthy oils. This then gets into our blood stream. Eczema is caused by systemic toxic overload and it's important that your daily moisturizer isn't contributing towards this. Let's break this down.

There is a popular product called Eucrisa that offers an eczema relief product. This product contains white petrolatum which is a by-product of petroleum which is created from crude oil. While the FDA has confirmed this product is safe it doesn't mean it won't make your eczema worse. It is saying "yes, this product won't kill you" but will it heal you? Absolutely not. There is a toxic ingredient in this product called propylparaben.

This ingredient has been found by the EWG (Environmental Working Group) to be an endocrine disrupter. Which in common language means that it messes with your hormones. Does this sound safe for eczema? Not to me. In the next section, you will learn about toxic ingredients to avoid in your everyday products.

Be sure to check all products you apply to your skin like makeup, lotions, and sunscreen.

Toxic Ingredients to Avoid

Try your best to avoid the ingredients you learn about on this page. Most of the ones we are going to go over lead to issues much more serious than eczema. I have used EWG, environmental working group, as my resource for this section of the book. I highly trust this company and hope you use their [website](#) as a tool. The first toxic substance we are going to talk about is BPA. This is found in plastic and aluminum cans. To avoid it make sure the label says BPA free. This is another reason why eating whole foods are better than processed because you don't have to worry about a sweet potato containing BPA but you have to worry about canned soup harming you. The next chemical is parabens. They are used in beauty products as a preservative and can really mess up your hormone balance. Moving on to phthalates which are found in some fragrances and negatively impact the reproductive system. One chemical I found particularly disturbing is actually found in Colgate Total toothpaste called triclosan. It really impacts the thyroid as well as hormones. Triclosan is also found in some antibacterial soaps, body wash, and even cutting boards.

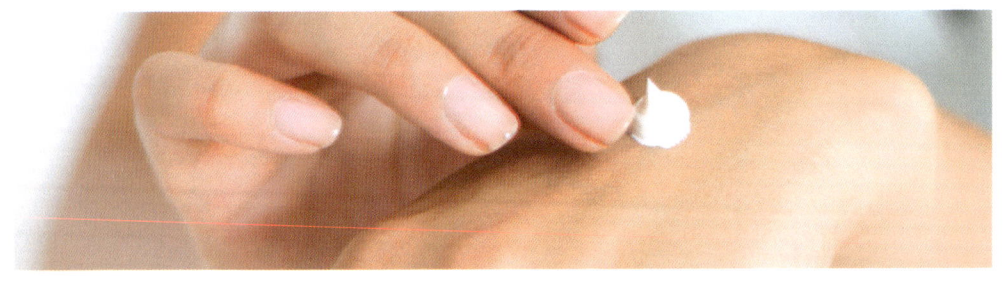

There are some products you need to be extra careful about and one of those is sunscreen. Very commonly sunscreens contain oxybenzone which can cause immune issues, organ toxicity, and reproductive problems. Another HUGE problem with most body products is that they usually contain fragrance which causes allergies, immune issues, and organ toxicity. While all the ones previously listed are in fact toxic I am going to list a few that I am not a fan of especially if you have eczema. These are not technically toxic but they sure don't make your skin heal. Try avoiding mineral oil, petroleum, lactic acid, any alcohols like stearyl or benzyl. The best idea is to make your own shampoo, body wash, and house cleaner. There are plenty of recipes online for that!

Topical Steroids & Antibiotics

I am sure that at sometime during your life with eczema you have sought the guidance of either a primary care doctor or a dermatologist. Unfortunately you were probably prescribed a topical steroid such as fluocinonide, hydrocortisone butryate or maybe prednicarvate. Your doctor may have taken another route and prescribed antibiotics such as flucloxacillin. This is actually pretty scary when you learn about the effects of these prescriptions on your sensitive body. For example, when you use topical steriods, your skin actually becomes much thinner. That is the least of your worries, though.

Long term use of topical steroids can leave the body dependent on them for "clear skin." I use quotes around clear skin because topical steroids actually do not heal the skin. I like to use a metaphor to explain this. Image that you live in a two story house. All of a sudden in your living room on the first floor you see a water stain on the ceiling. Over time this stain gets bigger and bigger. The stain on the ceiling represents your skin. The actual issue is that a pipe broke and it needs to be repaired. That is the same way that leaky gut needs to be repaired.

What do you do now? Well of course you call an expert. So you call up a ceiling repair person not a pipe repair person. If you are wondering why you would call a ceiling repair person instead of a pipe repair person than you understand how inaccurate it is to seek a dermatologist's help instead of someone who can help you repair the root cause issue. Back to the story, the ceiling repair person comes and sands down the places where the stain is and puts a little puddy down and then paints over the puddy. This is the same thing as topical steroids.
Has the leaky pipe been fixed? No.

I hope this story has helped you all understand what is happening when you use topical steroids. Unfortunately when you discontinue use of them they will cause severe damage. This is called topical steroid withdrawal or TSW. When you begin your natural healing journey you may experience TSW for a little while and it can be quite miserable but it does not last forever!

Topical Steroids & Antibiotics

On to discussing antibiotics and their massive affect on your long term health. This is a tricky subject because there is a time and a place for antibiotics. For example, serious bacterial inflections need to be taken care of using antibiotics.

In comparison to a bacterial infection, eczema is not nearly as severe. With that being said, using antibiotics could be the reason you have eczema in the first place. What do they do inside your body? Antibiotics eliminate all bacteria from your body, good and bad. If you never knew there was such a thing as good bacteria, then I am excited for you to learn!

Our whole bodies are covered in bacteria. Before you get scared, this is a great thing. For the most part this bacteria is good and helps you prevent getting sick. Fun fact, different parts of your body are home to different strains of bacteria. Even more fun, our bacteria changes from birth to adulthood! Birth is a critical aspect to "stocking" our bodies with beneficial bacteria. Research shows that babies who were born via c-section were at a higher risk for autoimmune conditions like eczema. This is because being born through the skin rather than naturally provides less diverse bacteria. While this is a relatively dense topic, the most important

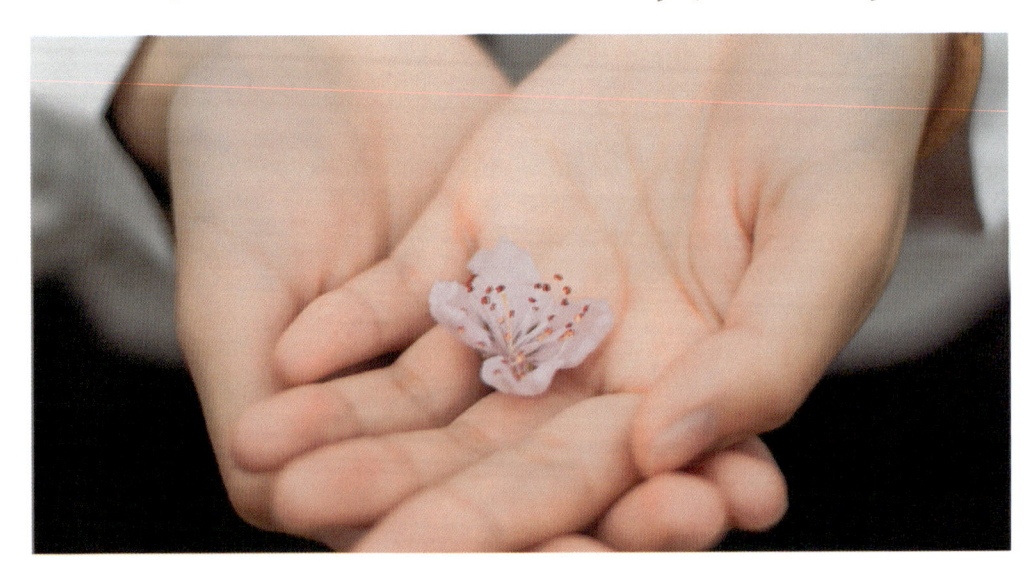

Topical Steroids & Antibiotics

thing for you to understand is that we need good bacteria on us and in us.

That means things like hand sanitizer, antibiotics, and harsh cleaning chemicals should only be used in serious cases. Hand sanitizer wipes your hands clean of good bacteria exposing your skin to a variety of harmful bacteria. For example if you use hand sanitizer then touch a door handle there is a greater chance of you getting sick from a bacteria you picked up. Being overly clean is not the life to live.

Things are starting to change but previously it was popularized in the media that clean is better. We thought that keeping ourselves in a bubble would prevent sickness. However, research shows that exposure to a wide range of bacteria is beneficial for us.

Stop fearing public transportation. It is a great place for us to meet a broad spectrum of bacterial strains. Going back to antibiotics, the same thing occurs but inside of our bodies. Antibiotics wipe our guts clean of all bacteria and leave us vulnerable to bad bacteria.

I can almost guarantee if you go on antibiotics you will end up with a yeast infection or a UTI because you are creating an environment those bacteria thrive in.

I am not saying that antibiotics are all bad. Just be careful and realize when it is beneficial.

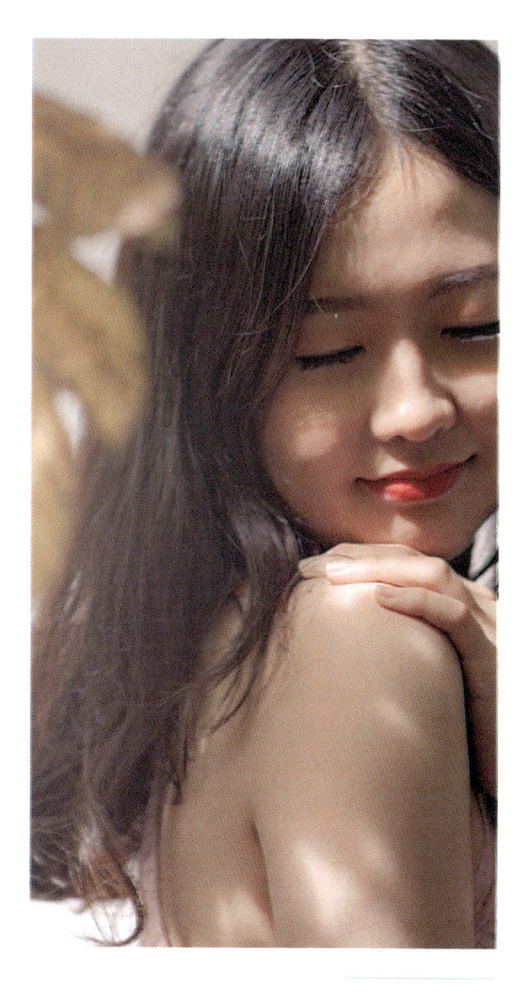

Eczema Healing Lifestyle Transformation © by Michelle Mills

Vital Nutrients for Healing

Omega 3 fatty acids are such a key aspect of healing. Inflammation is a huge part of many disorders and diseases which includes eczema.
Fats have two big categories which are unsaturated or saturated. Unsaturated fats are further broken down into two more sections being mono-unsaturated (an example is olive oil) and polyunsaturated.

At the moment nutrition experts only talk about two major polyunsaturated fatty acids which are omega-6 and omega-3. Examples of omega-6 are corn oil, sunflower oil, and almonds. Learning about nutrition can seem complicated. We are about to dive a little bit deeper and talk about how these fatty acids are metabolized.

Sometimes too much of a good thing can actually have the opposite affects. That is the case with omega-6 fatty acids. People, especially those that consume processed foods, are consuming far too many omega-6 fatty acids. Now we are going to really dive in.

Omega-6, without the presence of omega-3, can metabolize to be inflammatory. It can cause headaches, joint pain, or inflamed skin. We should strive to create a balance of omega-6 and omega-3. You do this through diet. Some great sources of omega-3 fatty acids include fatty fish like salmon, mackerel, or sardines.

There are also some plant-based foods like flaxseeds and chia seeds. This is where moderation and listening to your body will really benefit you. You should try to keep processed, packaged foods to a minimum. Start incorporating omega-3 fatty acid rich foods at least 3 times a week.

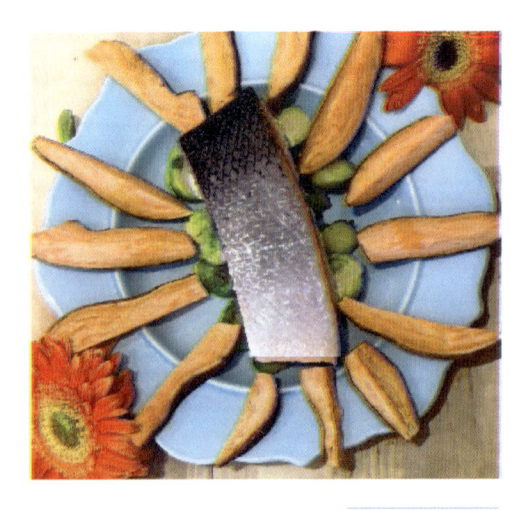

Eczema Healing Lifestyle Transformation ©
by Michelle Mills

Vital Nutrients for Healing

Vitamin D

Vitamin D is a nutrient that you can get from sun exposure, diet, or supplementation. The majority of the population isn't getting enough vitamin D so it is key that you understand how to get it into your life! When your body is healing it uses it's vitamin D supply up readily. That means you will need more vitamin D than the typical healthy person.

What are dietary sources of vitamin D? It is tricky because this nutrient is not abundant in foods. However, there are a few foods that at least can help you reach the level of vitamin D that you body needs as it is healing.

Mackerel is one example of a dietary source of vitamin D. For example, a 75g fillet of wild caught (always buy wild caught seafood) mackerel has about 350 IU of vitamin D. To put that into perspective, people should have around 400-800 IU daily. Another source of vitamin D is mushrooms.

Vitamin D comes in two different forms depending on if it's from a plant source or an animal source. Vitamin D3 comes from animal sources like the mackerel mentioned above. D3 can be used much faster than the plant based vitamin D called "D2." If you do not eat seafood, mushrooms or get much sun then you might want to look into taking a supplement. Make sure when you are looking for them that you notice if it is D3 or D2. You should chose one that has D3 and has about 1,000 IU.

Some brands of supplements that I approve of are: Life Extension, NOW, Garden of Life, or NatureWise. However, supplements change over time so be sure they don't contain "maltodextrin." You can go over to Google and look up bad ingredients in supplements. There is a really great list and it will give you many more examples.

Please check with your primary care doctor or dietitian before implementing any new supplements. Vitamin D is generally safe and doesn't typically interact with any medications. If you are getting vitamin D from the sun make sure to use proper protection, take polypodium (fern supplement), or limit sun expose to prevent skin cancer.

Vital Nutrients for Healing

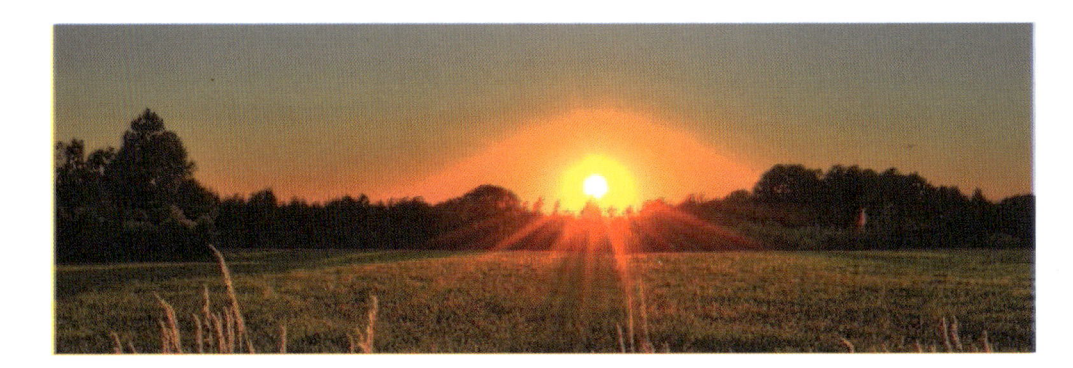

Amino Acids

In the supplement section of this book you will learn more about the best amino acids for healing. Amino acids are the building blocks of proteins. Proteins are used in our bodies in so many different ways. You may not have known this but hormones are actually proteins. Other functions of proteins include transporting nutrients, structure, and growth/maintenance of tissues. Amino acids are important for healing because of their ability to combine together to create these important proteins.

The goal is to give your body a broad range of amino acids through food sources for it to utilize in different ways. If you are plant based or vegan than you will find it interesting that quinoa is a complete protein. A complete protein means that it contains all of the essential amino acids our bodies can't produce themselves. Another wonderful plant based complete protein is hemp!

I recommend using a hemp protein powder as your vegan protein powder of choice. Hemp is high in iron which can help balance your immune system. I enjoy hemp protein added to my homemade sauces. You can even add it to banana nice cream which is essentially frozen bananas blended together.

Fun fact: l-lysine and l-proline help the body produce collagen.

Brands

There are a couple non toxic brands that I really love. The first brand I would like to mention is Australian Carob. They carry delicious "chocolate" that really isn't chocolate. Carob is a pod that comes off of trees that has a pulp in the center that can be dried and ground to create a lovely sweet treat. I recommend if you are in stage one to avoid chocolate, cocoa powder or cacao powder because it is likely to contain caffiene which can make eczema worse. Instead opt for carob powder or carob "chocolate" bars because it is absolutely eczema safe. Australian Carob also carries carob powder.

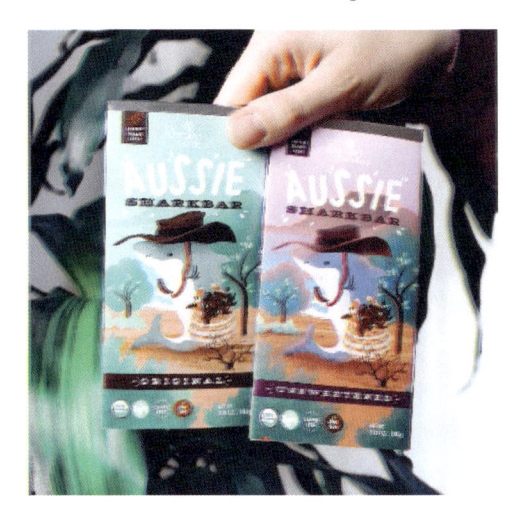

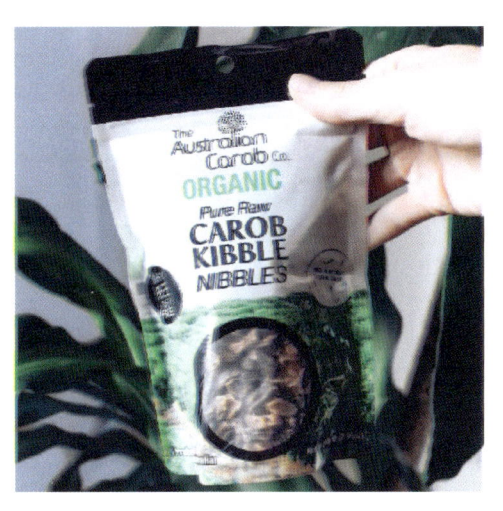

I use carob powder to create an amazing eczema safe dessert. I take frozen banana chunks, a plant based milk, carob powder and blend them together. It may take your brain a few tries to connect it to the taste of chocolate but after a while you won't miss chocolate. If you are an ice cream fan like me, then this is a perfect ice-cream-like treat! They also have a product called kibble. If you are someone who has to constantly chew something than this may really help you. Instead of gum, which may contain toxic ingredients, look into carob kibble. As far as flavors of the Sharkbars (carob bars) I highly recommend sticking to the plain unsweetened. Our bodies are very likely to have candida overgrowth. Any sweetener that can raise your glucose levels can feed candida.

Brands

If you follow me on Instagram you may have heard me rave about this next brand: Seed Phytonutrients. Not only does this brand's products come in an environmentally safe containers but the ingredients are non-toxic as well. I have never had hair products that actually cleanse my scalp, soften my hair, and leave it moisturized before. I highly recommend switching from the typical products like "Pantene" or "Garnier" to this brand to prevent toxic overload. Refer back to the to "Toxic Ingredients to Avoid" page as a guide for what to avoid in your day to day products.

There is an awesome brand worth mentioning with a massive product line of delicious food, Siete. While this isn't great for the early stages of healing, you will grow to love these products in stage 3 and forward. They have tortilla chips made out of cassava (which is gluten free because it isn't a grain, it is a root vegetable).

They come in all sorts of flavors like nacho and ranch. Get this, they are all void of FREDG foods. The nacho chips taste like cheese but with no cheese! They are flavored with a healthy cheesey tasting seasoning called nutritional yeast. They also have jars of queso and tortilla wraps! I love all of these products and feel safe eating them.

There are some really awesome brands of plant based yogurt too like Culina, Foragers, and Lavva. Culina is a great coconut yogurt that is packaged in a clay pot. This yogurt has clean ingredients but is also healthy for the environment. Foragers has a great unsweetened mylk and yogurt. Lavva is for less severe eczema because the base of it's yogurt is pili nut. It is very unusual but equally exciting. Be sure to read all the ingredients before you buy though!

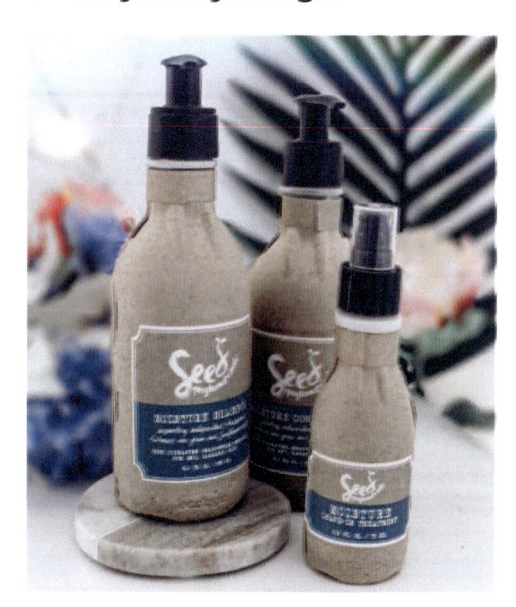

Kitchen Staples

How should you stock your pantry and fridge? What tools will help you lead a healthy life? Let's start with the fridge! Some staples you should always keep handy are flax oil, probiotics, salmon and cabbage. These are my top four power tools for health! Flax oil is rich in omega-3 which is anti-inflammatory. Probiotics stock your gut with healthy bacteria.

Cabbage can be added to any meal to create a mucus lining on your gut that prevents harmful substances from further creating leaky gut. Salmon is a powerhouse food meaning it is packed with amazing nutrients your body needs. Make sure your salmon is wild caught though!

Salmon provides your body with omega-3, iron, and b12 which aid your body in healing. The freezer is a wonderful thing! I highly recommend buying the majority of your vegetables and fruits frozen because they are picked ripe and frozen rather than picked under ripe and gassed to ripen. If you are conscious of the environment you could buy your produce from a farmers market or grow it yourself, then freeze it.

Frozen bananas are an excellent dessert. You can blend them to create an ice cream or slice them before freezing to make chocolate covered banana. To create a chocolate coating mix coconut oil and carob powder or chocolate chips (refined sugar free and dairy free). Melt the ingredients, cover the banana slices, and freeze again!

Moving on to the pantry I recommend always having white basmati rice, carob powder, cassava flour, and legumes. While I want your diet to be

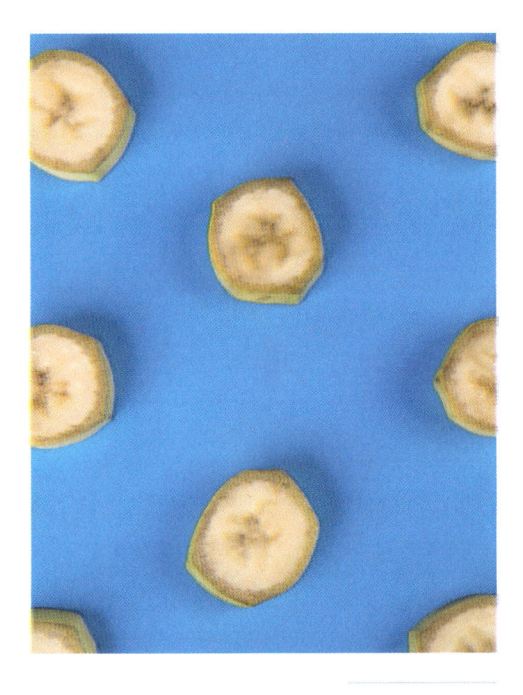

Kitchen Staples

mostly vegetables sometimes it is necessary to add calories using rice or legumes. Lentils and beans are legumes and can be very nutritional especially if you pressure cook them.

Going back to the banana ice cream, if you add carob powder to it you now have a chocolate ice cream with a slight licorice taste to it. I love adding carob to so many things because I have grown to love the taste! If you are like me and you get bored of foods often then the cassava flour can help you out! I love making homemade tortillas using cassava flour, water, and oil. Try googling a recipe, it is super simple. Add garlic powder and a little sea salt too.

There are some really fantastic tools that have made my life way easier when it comes to eating clean. The first is a ninja food processor which you can purchase on my shop on my website. I can easily blend my frozen bananas, make homemade cashew milk, homemade cashew butter, and yummy smoothies.

My next tool is very unusual. It is a large cloth or pillowcase. You use this to store your leafy greens in. It actually prevents them from going bad! It is an amazing trick I learned earlier in 2019 and has been working magic for me ever since. Make sure the cloth is tied so little air gets in. No more soggy lettuce!

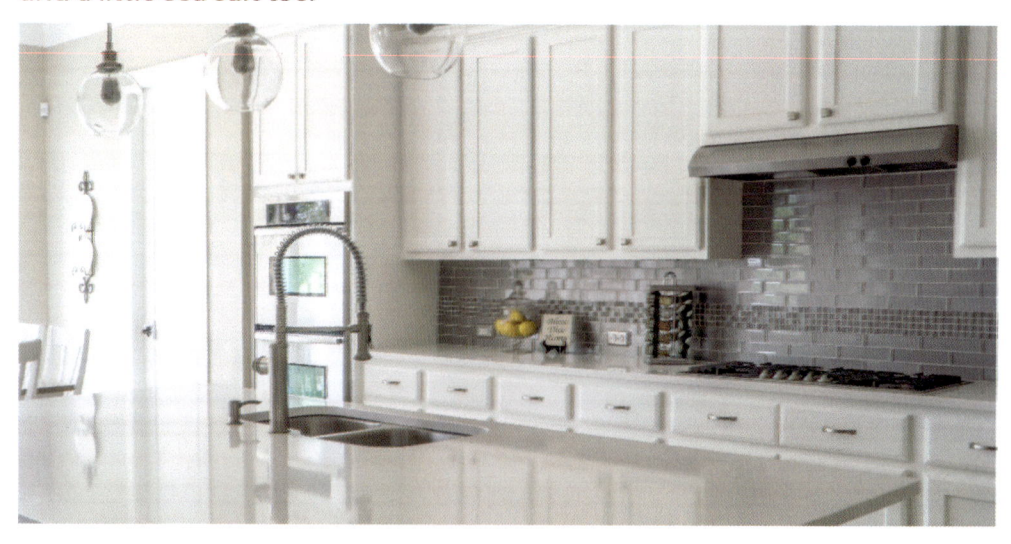

Eczema Healing Lifestyle Transformation ©
by Michelle Mills

www.coachmichellemills.com

Stage 1 Recipe

A Staple Recipe for Healing

I actually created this soup on accident. I didn't mean for this soup to be able to heal eczema as well as it does! I am so glad I did because I have had clients heal in half the time because of this soup. Fun fact about your body: your gut microbiome controls your cravings. If you crave sugar, that is a good indicator that you have candida. Since healing my gut I have been craving cabbage, beets, leeks, and bone broth. Sounds crazy but you will see. It is because the bacteria that lives in my gut, love these foods!

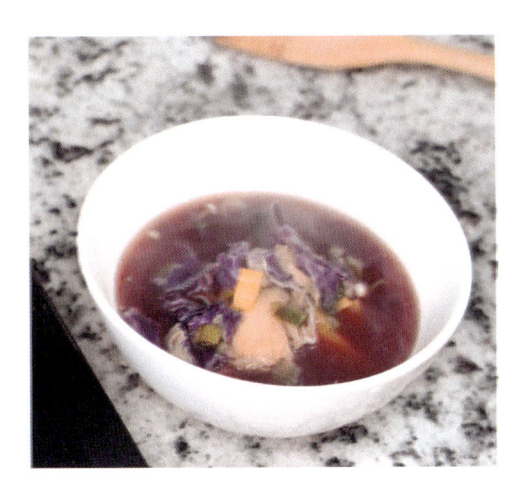

Gut Healing Super Soup

INGREDIENTS
1 cup bone broth
2 cup filtered water
2 cup of cabbage
1.5 cup of beets
0.25 cup leeks
0.5 cup of mushrooms
0.25 cup shaved brussel sprouts
Seasoning: garlic, sea salt, ginger, thyme

DIRECTIONS

1. Put bone broth + 1 cup of water in a pan, put on medium heat

2. Add cabbage and beets (they need to be cooked longest), cook for 7 minutes

3. Add a second cup of water + leeks, cook for 5 minutes or until cabbage is tender

4. Add in the seasonings (you choose how much to add based on taste)

5. Add the rest of the ingredients and cook until all ingredients are heated through

6. Serve

Bathing

Bathing can be a difficult task when you have eczema. We will address the different aspects of bathing like water temperature, filters, and what soaps to use. Have you ever noticed that you skin gets itchier or more red after bathing? There are many aspects that could be causing this. The frequency of bathing can even affect the health of your skin.

Imagine it is a cold winter night and you decide to take a hot shower. You will probably notice that hot water will make the skin feel numb while it is in contact with the skin. Once this stimulus is removed, the skin becomes extremely inflamed. This is actually because skin surface temperature greatly impacts flare-ups.

Recommendation:

Make sure to bathe with room temperature water or if that is uncomfortable during colder times, a little warmer than room temperature will be ok.

ESSENTIAL OILS

Lavender
Stress relief

Chamomile
Stress relief

Geranium
Skin health

Tea Tree
Antibacterial

Water Temperature

It is important that you control the temperature of your shower or bath. Research shows that quick changes in temperature can cause the skin to become aggitated.

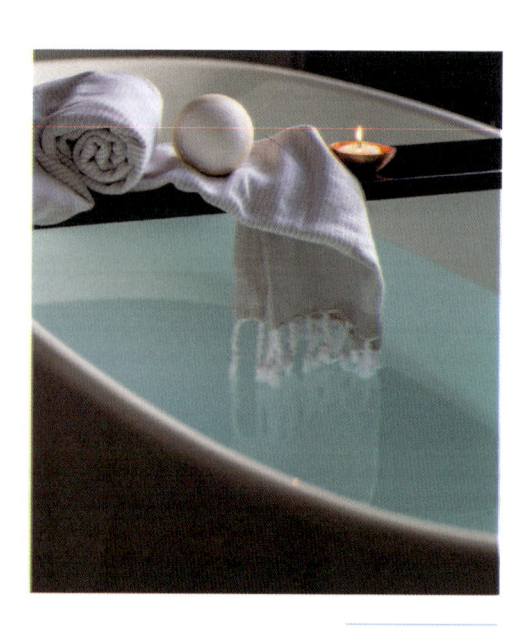

Eczema Healing Lifestyle Transformation ©
by Michelle Mills

Bathing

What to Add to Baths

There are many products on the market that claim to help eczema and this includes bath soaks. Severe eczema can be incredibly sensitive to chemicals and these products are likely to have tons of them. Do your research to make sure that whatever you are adding to your bath that it is safe to use. Try looking up the ingredients of your favorite bath bomb or bubble bath.

Recommendation:

You want to use products that have clean, non-toxic ingredients. Make sure to look up the ingredients on the Internet. Copy and paste them into Skin Charisma's ingredient analyzer to see if that product is safe. Stay away from any products that have a high risk.

I highly recommend using dead sea salt, essential oils, or bentonite clay in your baths. Dead sea salt is sea salt that comes from the Dead Sea which is in two countries which are Israel and Jordan. Dead sea salt contains a lot of minerals which can soak into the body through the skin. Think of your bath like a multi-mineral.

PRODUCT FAVORITES

Bath
Bentonite clay by Aztec Secret

Shampoo
Seed Phytonutrients

Acne Healer
Vitamin C Serum by Mad Hippie

Moisturizer
Shea butter by Alaffia

I have listed a few essential oils on the previous page and a quick explanation of how they help. You may be able to find dead sea salt with lavender essential oils together and that will work great. If you are adding your own essential oils to the bath, make sure they are organic and only use up to 10 drops.

As far as the bentonite clay, try using it by adding only 1/4 cup to your bath water. If the skin reacts well you can increase that to a cup per bath. Bentonite clay used to soothe my skin when it was at it's worst. I hope it is able to help you as well.

Bathing

Water Filters

Keep in mind that the water that flows through the pipes of your shower might not be the healthiest for your skin. If the water smells of chemicals like chlorine it is likely that you may need to invest in a shower head filter. Another problem that arises with eczema is that the skin is delicate and needs to maintain a balanced pH to prevent itch.

Recommendation:

Try using the internet to research the water in your city. If you suspect it may be filled with chemicals that are not great for sensitive skin then I would try finding a filter that fits your shower fixture. It may be a good idea to test the pH of your water as well. You may even consider changing your kitchen sink faucet out for a filtered one if you cook often. You don't want to cook with chemicals either.

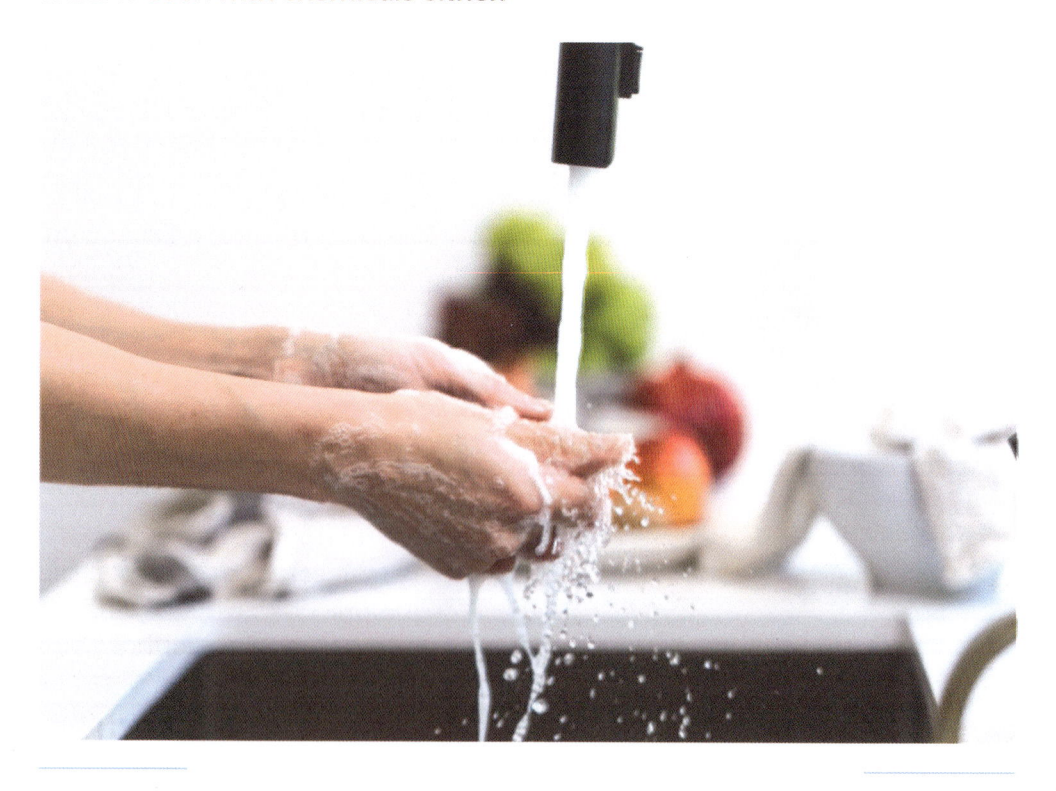

Bathing

Soaps, Shampoos, and More

It is critical that we know not only what chemicals are lurking in our food but also in our soaps. Our skin absorbs substances, good or bad, into our blood stream. It is important that the things our skin comes in contact with are healing rather than damaging. This goes for all individuals not just those with eczema. How can you tell what products are better than others? I would prefer if you all used products with simple ingredients but if you are unable to find that then I suggest using www.ewg.org to check the products for toxic ingredients as a start.

This is a website that is a data base of many popular products and the potentially harmful chemicals in them. For example I searched the popular shampoo brand: Pantene. It is given a score of "5" which means the ingredients aren't great but they don't cause cancer.

However, for those with eczema, any product with a score higher than 1 should not be used. Pantene shampoos contain harmful ingredients such as: fragrance, methylisothiazolinone, methylchloroisothiazolinone, cocamidopropyl betaine, sodium laureth sulfate, and sodium benzoate.

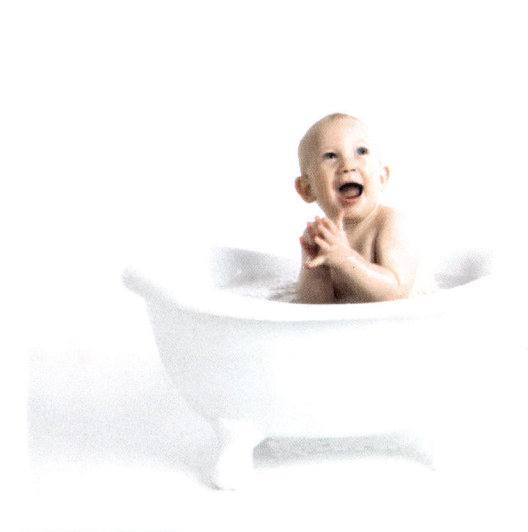

Recommendation:

Castile soap is a great replacement for hand and body soap. I highly recommend looking up a recipe for homemade shampoo also using castile soap. The recipes are simple and typically include essential oils, a little bit of oil like avocado oil and the castile soap.

Use the tips on this page for buying makeup, face wash, and even household cleaners. Lemon essential oil makes for a good cleaner.

Eczema Healing Lifestyle Transformation ©
by Michelle Mills

Your Home

Kitchen

Cooking

While cooking I recommend cooking with broths or filtered water. This is going to be a hard adjustment at first because most people commonly cook with oils. If you have to cook with oil I encourage you to use avocado oil because it is the most heat resistant. When oils like flax oil are heated, they oxidize very fast. Oxidation creates free radicals. Free radicals cause serious diseases like cancer. However, having a diet rich in vitamin C (papaya is high in vitamin c) can reverse this damage. Vitamin C is an antioxidant which means it repairs free radicals.

Living Space

Cleaning

It is recommended to steer clear of harsh chemical cleaners. There is a time and place for antibacterial cleaners and giving your home a general clean is not one of them. By removing all of the bacteria in your home, you are creating an environment where bad bacteria can run wild. Our homes are filled with good and bad bacteria. The good bacteria works to fight off bad. When you wipe the house clean of all bacteria, the good bacteria can no longer do it's job.

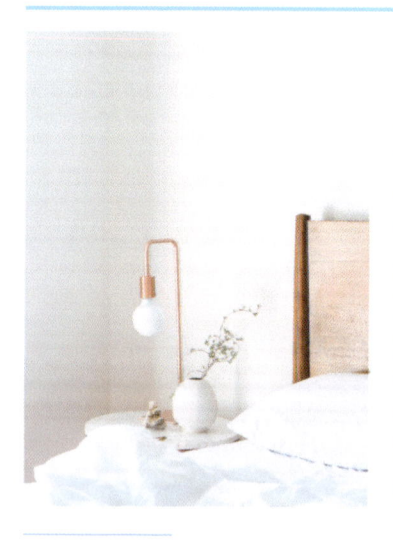

Bedroom

Sleeping

Creating a good sleep routine is extremely important for healing eczema. Your body heals the most during sleep. Try putting lavender essential oils on the sides of your neck close to your ears before bed. Lavender is known to help relax your body and help you prepare for sleep. Shut off the phone. Not only does your phone create distractions but studies show that the blue light that emits from your phone prevents your body from getting ready to sleep.

Social Life

How to Be Social with Eczema

Eczema is a tough thing to go through emotionally and personally. It becomes harder when you try to balance a social life along with it. It is important to be social to reduce stress and feel support. I will teach you ways to alter your social life so you can heal your skin but have fun with friends.

Altering Your Social Life

Instead of doing the usual coffee date or lunch date try speaking up and suggesting things to do that are not related to eating. I suggest going for a walk, going to the beach, going to the zoo, or roller skating. Being active with your friends is a great way to bond and get in your daily exercise. If you have to go out to eat for some reason speak up and suggest places that accomdate the eczema diet. I like to ask people to go to juice bars with me to get a green juice. Another great tip for eating out is to use Happycow.com as a tool to find vegan restaurants. While the eczema diet is not vegan it helps finding places that are already egg free and dairy free. The best bet is to find a raw vegan restaurant. Typically these places are completely eczema friendly with items that avoid FREDG foods. You may also be able to find decadent desserts from these places as well!

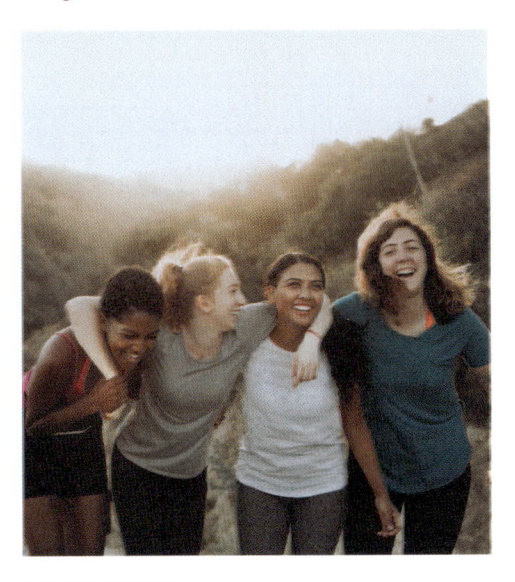

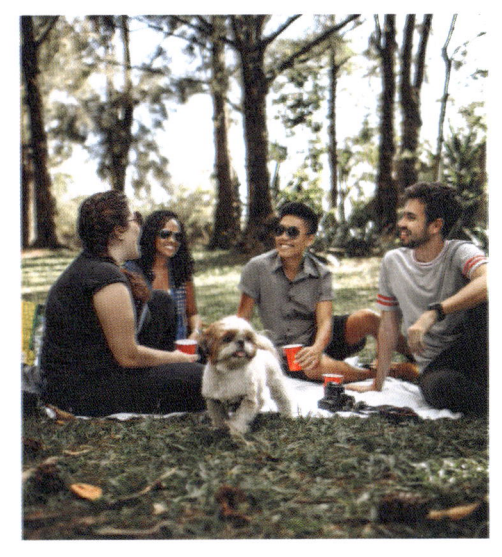

Social Life

Dating/Relationships
Eczema can make your love life pretty difficult. If you are going through very severe eczema your partner will have to be very patient. If your partner is causing you stress I recommend taking a break from the relationship until you heal.

If you are dating, try looking for people that make you feel good about yourself. Try finding someone who is caring and compassionate. A selfish partner is likely to lead to a toxic relationship and worsening eczema. It is very important you have support during this journey. Going on dates might be tricky but use the advice from the Altering Your Social Life section and suggest "non-food" dates like going hiking. Make sure you wear clothing on your dates that won't hurt your eczema. It is better to wear something that makes you feel comfortable rather than impress another person. Imagine wearing something too hot or too itchy and feeling like you want to tear your skin off. You are likely to come across very uncomfortable to your date. Be yourself. Be honest. I always recommend to my clients that it is better to be completely up front with your partner about your skin. Say "I have an autoimmune disorder called eczema and I am healing it naturally."

Surviving The Workplace
Many individuals end up taking time off of work to heal their skin if it is very severe. If this is not an option for you, then I have a few tips for surviving the work place. I recommend explaining to your employer that you have eczema, it is not contagious, and you are treating it. If you feel close to a coworker seek support from them. I also highly suggest meal prepping on the weekend and bringing your own food to work. White basmati rice is an example of one thing you can meal prep. Papaya cut up into cubes or slices as a snack helps too. It is very important that you make time in your schedule to make your own food. Prioritize making dinner after work. You do not want to end up having no other choice but to eat out. If you do eat out "make-your-own" salad bars are great and so are Japanese restaurants. You can eat salmon sashimi and miso soup from there.

Outdoors

You probably would have never guessed that being outside is important to your health. With that being said being outside in a polluted area sometimes does more harm than good. In this section, I am going to tell you the positives of being outside. Going back to the conversation about the bacteria that live on our body, did you know that bacteria are all around us as well? Activities like gardening, being barefoot in the sand, or playing in a grassy area will expose you to some of the best bacteria for healing.

The beach is a holy grail for healing because of the sand and the ocean. The ocean is home to so many amazing bacteria that will help your skin heal. If you are not close to a beach then try to start gardening. Try not to wear gloves because the goal is to expose your skin to the soil. It's time to get dirt under your nails! If you do not have space to garden then go to a public park and get your bare feet onto the grass. This is like taking a probiotic supplement but through the skin! Getting outdoors will allow you to get sunlight (natural vitamin D) and promote physical activity. Physical activity lowers stress hormones, lowers your blood sugar, and gets you sweating. Sweat has antibacteria properties which in turn help your skin!

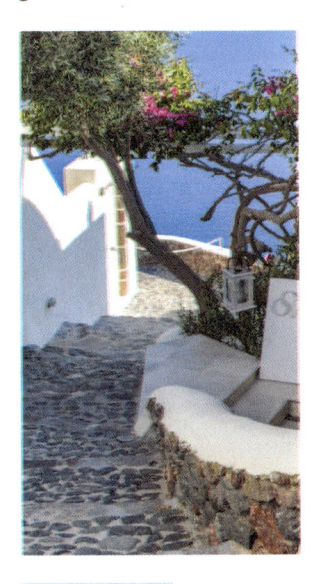

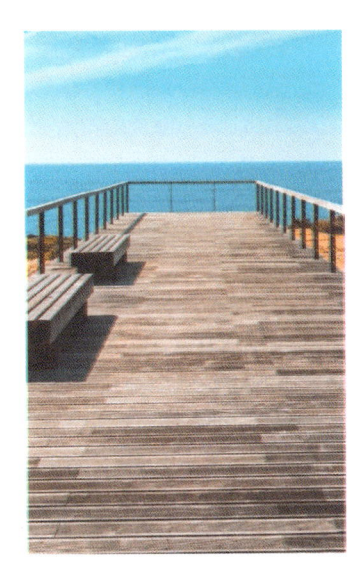

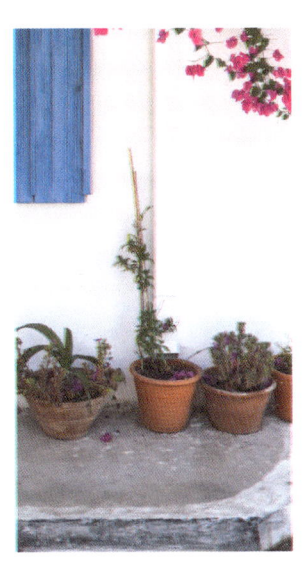

Mentality & Faith

The blue zones describe areas of the world where people live to be very old. These civilazations consistently have people reach old age in a healthy way. These places also have a very little incidence of autoimmune disorders. That means something about their way of living prevents problems like eczema. What is it that they do so right? It is a combination of lifestyle, diet, faith, and family.

The best part of the blue zones is that these individuals achieved health with very little income. They often walk long distances to purchase food (typically up and down hills), they have active jobs like farming, and never go out to eat because they live more simple lives. When society "progressed" into having fast food, packaged goods, and mass farming, our health declined as a result. It may not be realistic to mimic the lives of the ones that live in blue zones but you can adopt some of their habits. The one, in particular, I want to address in this section of the book is faith.

One commonality among people that live in the blue zones is that they have strong faith. It doesn't matter if you believe in religion or just spirituality. Connecting yourself to something bigger leads to something beautiful. This may seem like a hard time in your life but there are still so many great things happening in your life to be grateful for. Life, in general, is something you should find love and gratitude for. We are able to breathe air, love, heal, and impact others around us. It is time for you to spread love. Go out of your way to do something nice for another person and see how beautiful you start to feel. Healing isn't just physical. During this journey strive to heal your mentality.

I always found that sleep meditations or morning affirmations were very helpful. If I had trouble sleeping, I would go to YouTube and listen to a sleep meditation by "Dauchsy." It is uplifting, calm, and guides you through breathing exercises. Another thing I still do is listen to morning affirmations.

There is magic in using the words "I am..." and in particular you should repeat these: I am healthy. I am determined. I am beautiful. I am thankful.

Eczema Healing Lifestyle Transformation ©
by Michelle Mills

Moisturizing

Wow this is such an important topic! So many people are making massive mistakes when it comes to moisturizing their skin. Some people over moisturize and others put toxic creams on their skin. I have a YouTube video talking about the 5 best moisturizers that might be helpful for you to watch. I also have another video explaining the five worst as well. These videos are a good starting point but let's go deeper by addressing how often you should moisturize your skin. The short answer is It depends on how severe your skin is but chances are you are probably over moisturizing your skin.

If you have severe eczema that is so dry that it cracks or bleeds then you should moisturize once in the morning and once at night. If you go to work you can bring emergency cream but make sure to only use it if you skin is about to crack. When you over moisturize your skin you are stopping your body from producing it's own oil which will help your skin repair long term. If your eczema is in stage 2 then I encourage you to use moisturizer less and less. Start off by twice a day then in a week move to once a day. After time you will no longer need it.

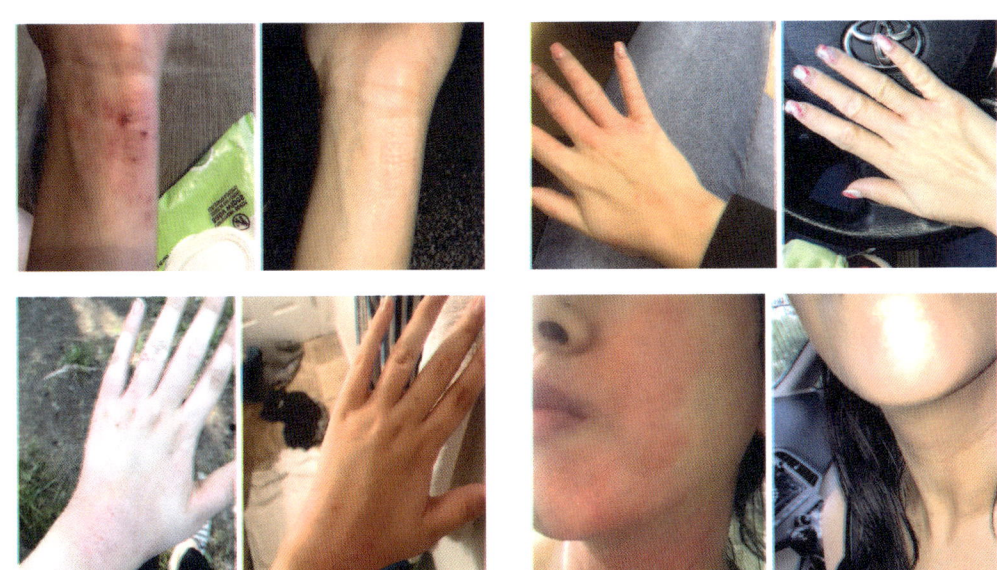

Eczema Healing Lifestyle Transformation ©
by Michelle Mills

Fad Diets & Eczema

There are a lot of different diets that people claim help people with eczema. There are some people that have healed through a vegan diet and others that have healed through a carnivore diet. There are many resources on the internet with lists of food that make eczema worse. I get a lot of questions about this because it causes a lot of confusion. My best piece of advice is to find someone you trust to provide you with diet guidance or do the research yourself.

If you decide to do it yourself you have to make sure that your sources are credible. You also should be aware that people are paid to release false claims based on "research." Big companies like Nestle or Kraft Heinz Company can and will pay scientists to write papers that "prove" claims like food safety.

A huge example is Monsanto who paid researchers to disprove "Roundup", a weed killer, is cancerous. As of 2019, they are actually facing a lawsuit because of this information. A safe and credible source I like to use NCBI. com to read research papers. Even if you use a credible source like NCBI, it is still important to read many papers with good supporting evidence.

I did months of research to develop the diet that I coach my clients with. Many people wonder what sets my diet apart. The difference is the research and speed of healing. The reason why fad diets like the ketogenic, paleo, or carnivore diets might work is that it pushes people to eat clean whole foods. When you get away from horrible processed foods there is great potential for your skin to heal if it isn't severe.

I did research on how to heal leaky gut, detox the liver, and balance the immune system through food and supplements. The vegan diet potentially can work but it takes nearly triple the time and doesn't promote gut healing unlike the diet I designed. With that being said I have helped coach people who have chosen a vegan diet for ethical reasons. I think the biggest benefit of my program and specialized diet is that you get to work with me closely as a coach to encourage you. Eczema healing can be lonely.

Sleeping

Gloves, gloves, gloves. The one thing that saved my skin during sleep is gloves. I wore a pair of soft cotton gloves to bed when I was healing my skin to prevent myself from tearing my skin to pieces! If I forgot my gloves I was sure to itch my skin in my sleep and cause it to spread. It is so important that you develop a night time routine. Destressing before bed will lessen the itching during sleep. I recommend taking a bath before bed, putting lavender essential oil behind your ears, and deep breathing. Put your electronic devices on the other side of the room and read a book before you sleep. Don't forget to take a glycine before bed as well. It promotes healthy sleep. Desperate times call for desperate measures. One of my clients put an ankle weight around their wrist at night to weigh their arms down. She found that she would wake herself up before she would start itching. Be careful with this method you could potentially harm yourself but I thought it was worth mentioning. One last piece of sleeping advice is to keep your room cool at night because heat can cause inflammation in the skin. Sleeping can be one of the hardest tasks when you have severe eczema but is one of the most important aspects of sleep. Take care of yourself and allow yourself time to get plenty of rest. Remember, health is wealth.

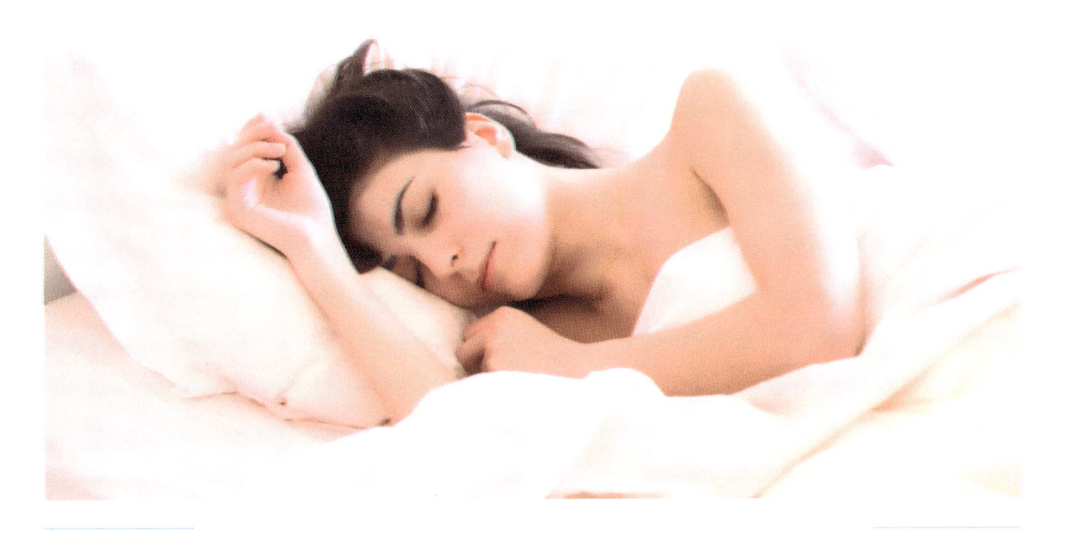

FREDG Foods Charts

Gluten

As a reminder, gluten is found in some grains. There are many foods that are made using grains like bread, pancakes, dosa, cakes, cookies, pasta, and pastries. You will need to read the ingredients if you chose to buy packaged foods instead of eating at home. Use the chart below to avoid grains that have gluten.

Grains Containing Gluten

Wheat

Barley

Rye

Semolina

Farro

Spelt

Malt

Durum

Unusual Sources of Gluten

Beer

Sauce

Dressing

Gravy

Gluten-free & Eczema

Rice

Gluten-free Oats

Quinoa

Buckwheat

Alternative Flour Options

Cashew flour

Cassava flour

Chickpea flour

Coconut flour (stage 2+)

Sweet Potato flour

Bob's Red Mill 1 to 1 Gluten-free

Almond flour (stage 3)

Eczema Healing Lifestyle Transformation ©
by Michelle Mills

FREDG Foods Charts

Dairy

True dairy is any product created from the milk of an animal. This can be found in so many products ranging from baked goods like cake to drinks like lattes. Lactose is a sugar found in dairy which causes leaky gut. I don't advice you to consume lactose free milk like Lactaid because it is highly processed. Stick to plant-based milk products you make at home.

Foods Containing Dairy

Cake

French Toast

Lattes, Macchiatos, Cappuccinos

Most Chocolate

Cheese, Yogurt, Sour Cream

Some Soups

Unusual Sources of Dairy

Some Supplements

Salad Dressing

Alcohol (cream liquors)

Artificial Sweetener (Equal)

Chip Dip

Dairy-free Replacements

Rice Milk

Cashew Milk/Cheese

Almond Milk/Cheese

Oat Milk

Flax Milk

Dairy-Free Brands

Siete

Parmela Creamery

Australian Carob

So Delicious

Good Karma

FREDG Foods Charts

Sugar

Refined sugar hides in many processed foods. Manufacturers can get away with calling it by many names. For example, you may see the word "dextrose." I also advise against products that contain artificial sweeteners. While they are deemed safe by the FDA, they often contribute greatly to autoimmune disorders caused by leaky gut.

Avoid These

Corn syrup

Brown sugar

Beet sugar

Cane sugar

Jaggery

Slenda

Equal, Nutrasweet

Sweet 'N Low, Aspartame

Dextrose, Maltodextrin

Turbinado

Malt syrup

Rice syrup

Confectioner's sugar

Safe for Stage 1

Maple syrup

Safe for Stage 2

Maple syrup

Stevia

Monk Fruit

Safe for Stage 3

Maple syrup

Coconut nectar, coconut sugar

Stevia

Monk Fruit

Note: Raising your blood sugar via dates, maple syrup, or fruit can cause inflammation. Only use sweeteners in moderation.

Eczema Healing Lifestyle Transformation © by Michelle Mills

FREDG Foods Charts

Eggs

I wanted to share with you what foods are commonly made with eggs. Some of these foods are more common to the United States so if you are not familiar with them don't worry. Eggs are used in a lot of dishes to bind substances together. For example, you use egg to bind food to the breading like making chicken tenders breaded with bread crumbs.

Common Foods with Eggs

Waffles

Bread, French toast

Frittata

Casseroles

Macaroons

Baked goods

Mayonaise

Coleslaw

Chicken salad

Potato salad

Fried rice

Breaded/fried foods

Quiche

Egg Replacements

Chia seeds - baked goods

Flax seeds - baked goods

Banana - baked goods

Applesauce - baked goods

Tofu + Black Salt (don't use black salt in stage 1 or 2) - tastes like egg to make scramble or sandwich

Conclusion

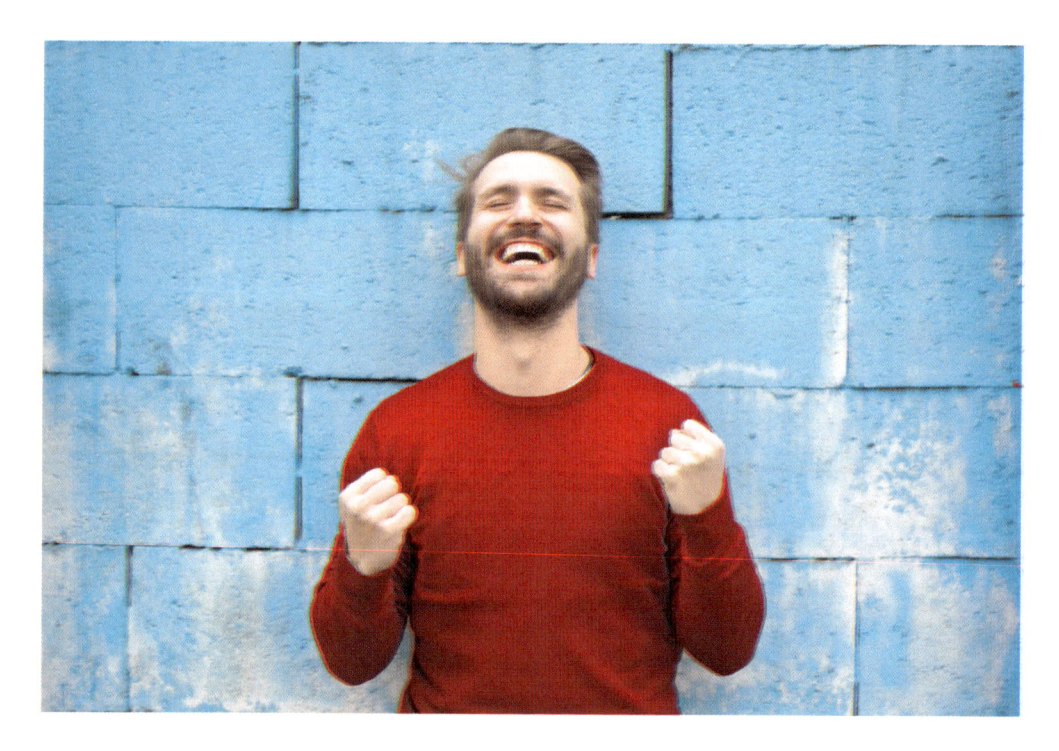

Congratulations! Finishing this book is one step of many towards your healing. Implement what you learned and teach others. Spread love and support for others who have eczema. You know how hard it is. We are a community that stands strong together. We are fighting against a society that believes in a magic pill (or cream for that matter). You are part of something much bigger. We can make a change and guide people away from topical steroids, antibiotics, and immune shots. Money follows the crowd and we are the crowd. I wish you the best of luck healing and once again if you need my help message, email, or join my Facbook support group. I have made it through this and you will too. One final piece of advice I can offer is to not be afraid to seek help. Eczema can lead to disordered thinking, stress, and anxiety. If you are dealing with such things please meet with a counselor to help you work through those thoughts. Your life is important to me and other eczema survivors. Once you get through this you can inspire others! Take care, ezcema friend.

- Thank You -

This journey is far from easy and I am blessed to be able to work with individuals to help them along this journey. I want to thank my parents for believing in me. They were patient with me as I learned how to heal my own eczema. I am thankful to be able to share my knowledge with you, the reader.

Thank you for reading.